Kelee® *Meditation*

Free your Mind

Ron W. Rathbun

KELEE® MEDITATION
Free your Mind

This book is an original publication of Quiescence Publishing

PRINTING HISTORY
Quiescence Publishing first edition / September 2012
Quiescence Publishing second edition / July 2013

www.thekelee.com
ISBN: 978-0-9841608-3-9

PRINTED IN THE UNITED STATES OF AMERICA

Contents

Kelee meditation

is a practice ...

that you can learn to do

on your own!

Kelee meditation is a practice that you can learn to do for yourself via learning the anatomy of the Kelee itself. The Kelee's reference points are a guide to help you understand how to do this meditation. When you learn how to get out of the brain and into your mind, you will learn how to still your thoughts. Stilling your mind will teach you how to let go of what hurts you, and open to what helps you.

Kelee meditation only takes 5 – 10 minutes twice a day and when it becomes a daily habit, you will watch your life change in an amazing way, right before your eyes. Then you will know for yourself, that your life is in your own hands, when you can still your mind to accept it.

Part One
Kelee Meditation: Preparation

The Lesser Kelee ⟶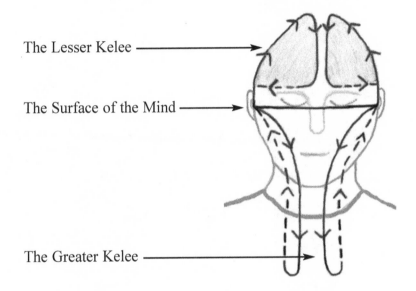

The Surface of the Mind ⟶

The Greater Kelee ⟶

The Kelee and its Major Points of Reference

*F*ind a place in your home
that can become a sanctuary
from the cares and worries
of the outside world.

*Find a place to do your practice that is peaceful
and conducive to tranquillity.*

A quiet place is a sanctuary for your soul. Find a comfortable place to do your meditation, but do not restrict doing your practice only to your favorite place. If you feel secure meditating only in your sanctuary, it will become a ritual and limit your ability to practice anywhere. A routine is good as long as it is not limiting.

The biggest distraction while meditating will be noise. When you can detach from sense consciousness in a noisy place, your mind gains strength and becomes more focused. As you progress in letting go of your senses, you will be able to do your practice almost anywhere.

Free your mind from the outside world.

Before you do your practice, turn off all outside distractions such as radios, television sets, phones, and pagers. Use your answering machine to help organize your time, do not become a slave to technology.

Inform anyone who may interrupt you that this is your quiet time and to please not disturb you. When those around you begin to see the benefits from your calmness, they will learn to honor your request for quiet time.

*M*editate in the silence of the morning
before the activity of your mind begins,
and in the quiet of the evening
before becoming too tired.

*Meditate early in the morning
when the outside world is quiet.*

Practice meditation before your mind becomes active and invents excuses why other things need doing. The intellect can think of countless reasons why you do not have time to meditate; this is when you need to meditate the most! Once patterns in your brain start moving, they do not like to stop. Behavior patterns feed off movement of energy and do not want to relinquish control to your conscious awareness and be still.

Do you ever notice when you are thinking, it is as if there are two of you? One part is your brain i.e., intellect which likes to think and do, and the other part is your mind i.e., spirit which likes to experience and feel. Your mind is the detached, nonlinear part of your spiritual essence whose sense of accomplishment comes from simple enjoyment and inner contentment rather than doing things at any cost.

Meditate in the evening before you get too tired.

If you are a person who is exhausted at the end of the day, do your practice earlier in the evening before you get too weary. It is a bad habit to meditate and fall asleep. You are training your mind to become still, not to sleep. In the early stages of learning to meditate, it is very important to make a clear distinction between sleep and stillness. If you are not sure if you fell asleep or if you were meditating, examine how you feel when you come back to full awareness. If you are groggy, you were drifting into sleep. If you are alert and wide-awake upon return, you were meditating properly.

*Sitting in meditation
with your spine erect
is not the mark of an enlightened man
but one who is diligent and aspiring
to reach enlightenment.*

Proper posture is good discipline.

Sitting with your spine erect is correct posture, a good habit and the way to teach your mind the difference between meditation and nodding off or wandering without control. When your spine is erect, it signals your mind to remain in a relaxed state but not to sleep. If you lie down to meditate, your brain will probably signal your awareness to become drowsy, because this is the position you assume when you sleep. You already know how to sleep; you are learning to meditate. Sleep is permitting your awareness to spread out into unconsciousness, while Kelee meditation is allowing your conscious awareness to be in a state of one-pointed stillness without drifting.

*Sitting in a comfortable position is
the absence of distraction.*

It is not necessary to sit in a cross-legged or lotus position to practice Kelee meditation. It is perfectly acceptable to sit in a chair with your feet flat on the floor.

Balance your head in an effortless-effort position.

How you hold your head during meditation is very important. It can be a major distraction if it falls forward or backward, straining your neck muscles. Tilt your head forward and back a few times until you feel the position where your head is balanced naturally; this is the "effortless-effort" position. Once again, this is simply basic good posture.

*The breath
is to the physical
what silence
is to the spiritual: essential.*

Breathing is a natural function of being.

Breathing is essential for the physical body, but to access deeper states of mind, the breath must be allowed to be at a resting state. If you cannot let go of focusing on the breath, you will not be able to get out of sense-consciousness which keeps you in the brain. In Kelee meditation you simply breathe normally. As you detach from sense consciousness, your breathing will naturally move to a resting state. In this state of being, your body's aging process slows, which ultimately lengthens your life.

What to do with your hands?

It seems many people do not know what to do with their hands. It is not necessary to have a special position for your hands other than being relaxed and comfortable. I prefer to have my hands resting in my lap palms up, simply because it feels natural. Once again, the goal is to be free of sense-consciousness distractions.

Being physically comfortable is necessary
to do Kelee meditation correctly.

Wear clothing that will not distract you. If your clothing is too tight, your brain will register tension, which will distract your attention and make it difficult to calm down. If you cannot let go of sense consciousness, physical tension will not allow you to drop into deeper states of mind.

The eyes are the windows to the soul,
but one does not have to be
looking through them
all of the time.

Relax and allow your eyes to rest during your practice.

It is a common problem to have difficulty closing your eyes during your practice; tension from thought prevents the eyes from relaxing. After all, your eyes are at the surface of your mind, the central location where thoughts are generated. Typically, eyestrain is caused because you work too long and fill your life with more activities than you need to. Any time you cross the line of moderation, something in your life will suffer.

When you begin to meditate, you may be startled to realize how much stress your eyes are carrying. When you exert excessive analytical energy at the surface of the mind, your eyes can become overworked. Eyestrain during meditation can be a major distraction. Relaxing your conscious awareness and calming the surface of your mind relieves considerable pressure from the eyes and is physically and mentally therapeutic.

If you are unable to softly and gently close your eyes, you are not relaxed and light coming from the outside world will tend to draw your awareness to the surface of your mind and the thinking process. Eyestrain is a physical form of tension, which will not allow your conscious awareness to drop into your greater Kelee, where detachment and stillness of the mind are found.

With practice over time, all tension problems associated with the eyes can be solved. Eyestrain comes from a mind that strains; relax and the windows to your soul will begin to open and close effortlessly.

*Calming the brain
relaxes
the physical body.*

When brain function calms, the physical body relaxes.

When thought activity in your brain races, it does not allow you to calm your conscious awareness and it is impossible to relax your physical body. It is of great benefit to detach from sense consciousness to ease tension in the physical body. The world of sense consciousness is filled with stress, i.e., glare to the eyes, loud noises to the ears, anything that is offensive to the physical senses. The muscle structure of the body works from tension, but if the muscular system is not allowed to rest, it grows fatigued. Finding moderation in the mind is vital. The key is quieting the mind and not inflicting undue pressure on the body.

In this practice, you ultimately want to be aware of nothing—complete stillness of mind without the distractions of the outward senses and body.

Conscious awareness changes as it moves from an intellectual function at the surface of the mind into the timeless realm below the surface in the greater Kelee. All on the planet who are seeking spiritual fulfillment are looking for this realm or state of mind, and it is within everyone. It is found by exploring your Kelee and your true spiritual nature. It all starts with a quiet state of mind, and evolves into states of perception that free the mind to move deeper and deeper to that which is the purest state anyone can be—complete self-understanding and that of absolute love.

A conscious awareness
is knowing
what you are doing
while you are doing it.

Locating your conscious awareness on command.

When you know how, you can learn to feel your conscious awareness on command. If I ask you to feel your fingertips, your conscious awareness will automatically go to them. If I say bring your conscious awareness to the top of your head, your awareness will go there. Where you direct your attention is where your conscious awareness will be.

Step One: For about two minutes, bring your conscious awareness to the top of your head and allow it to relax down through both hemispheres of the brain down to the surface of the mind. *Feeling* your conscious awareness as a horizontal plane relaxing through the brain to the surface of the mind.

Superimposed over the right and left hemispheres of the brain are numerous compartments of tension. These compartments are responsible for much of the chatter in your mind. When this chatter is calmed, you will be calmed. **Step One** of Kelee meditation will dissipate these compartments of mental tension over time.

The relaxed energy of your conscious awareness moving over compartments is like water moving over dirt clods. You will break down these compartments until one day they are completely washed away. With practice, you will be amazed at how your mind will change. However, you will never know until you practice.

*Kelee meditation
opens your mind
to one of the greatest gifts
you can give yourself,
experiencing silent miracles in your life.*

Kelee meditation becomes self-explanatory through the enlightenment of your own mind.

As the chatter in your brain diminishes, your sensitivity to subtle energy increases. As you sharpen and focus your conscious awareness, you become aware of the electrochemical energy of your mind. You begin to sense the difference between hard analytical energy and the soft subtle energy that allows your conscious awareness to feel with greater clarity.

Step Two: When your conscious awareness is relaxed at the surface of your mind, you can descend into the greater Kelee—the entrance to your soul. Remain at a still point in your greater Kelee for about three minutes and then come back to the surface of your mind to full awareness.

As you drop, within the greater Kelee, mind function detaches from brain function and an independent observer emerges. This independent observer is composed of subtle energy and becomes the light of awareness illumining the darkness of negative emotion trapped in your Kelee.

When your conscious awareness no longer has to fear, it opens. When fear does not feed fear, you do not mentally feed fearful dysfunction; fear must have energy to survive. When negative emotion is not given energy, it dissipates and your overall vibration is transformed, changing your whole being.

As you become aware of who you are without fear, a miracle begins to happen: you feel your true spiritual nature appear from within.

*The surface of the mind
is where
brain function
meets mind function.*

The surface of the mind is the primary reference point in Kelee meditation.

If you pay attention to where you understand what you are reading right now, you will notice that you can feel where your thinking is located; it is a horizontal plane of electrochemical energy exactly at eye level. This is the proverbial and literal surface of your mind. This plane of energy is where brain function and mind function meet. The area on top of the surface has to do with thinking and the area below the surface has to do with feeling. If I say *feel the surface of your mind*, your awareness automatically goes there. Being aware of this reference point, and the ability to calm it, will open the entrance to your heart and soul.

Setting your mind's biological clock.

Setting your biological clock is as simple as instructing yourself to return to full awareness at a specific time; your mind will automatically call you back. This inherent timing mechanism is what many people use to wake up at a certain time each morning or what signals them to go to bed each evening. Your biological clock is a useful tool when you are in deeper states of meditation, below the surface of your mind, where linear time does not exist. In the greater Kelee there is no sensation of time, so the biological clock is needed to bring you back, which in this practice occurs after approximately three minutes.

Note: After you have been practicing for a while, setting your biological clock becomes an automatic response as a natural part of Kelee meditation.

The heart
of Kelee meditation
is found below the surface of the mind
in the greater Kelee.

Allowing your conscious awareness
to drop into the entrance to your soul.

Within all of us is a field of electrochemical energy that is the entrance to our soul. It is where your conscious awareness is free from the constraints of the brain network. In this field of energy, you will find the key to unlock the chains that bind you in habitual patterns.

The foremost component of Kelee meditation is in learning to calm your conscious awareness and allow it to relax down below the surface of your mind until you come to a natural resting point in your greater Kelee. When you reach this resting point, keep all of your awareness together and remain quiet as you can for about three minutes. One of the first observations you will make when doing this part of Kelee meditation is, *If I am down here, what's up there?* The minute you have this thought your conscious awareness will return you to the surface of your mind. With practice, you will learn to be still in your greater Kelee, free from the distractions of the outside world.

Note: Do not look around with your mind's eye when in your greater Kelee, because you will start to think and return to the surface of your mind where thinking occurs.

Once again, **Step Two** of Kelee meditation is to remain at a still point in your greater Kelee for about three minutes and then come back to the surface of your mind, to full awareness.

As with any thing, practice makes perfect. When you have attained this form of perfection, you have done something truly remarkable.

*Upon returning to full awareness
from meditation,
review your practice through introspection,
then take time for contemplation.*

The Three Principles of Kelee Meditation

1. *Meditation.* Do Kelee meditation. The hardest thing about Kelee meditation is to simply do it. Kelee meditation takes approximately ten minutes twice a day, which is only one percent of your day. Never will you put so little into something and receive so much in return. Kelee meditation is a maintenance program for cleansing the mind and at the same time awakening the soul to enlightenment.

2. *Introspection.* This is **Step Three** of Kelee meditation. Upon returning from meditation, review what you remember from your practice for about five minutes.

The introspection portion of Kelee meditation is for retrospective observational purposes, to evaluate your meditation. The time you devote to introspection will teach you a great deal about who you are. If you are visualizing, observing, or planning while meditating, you are thinking and not doing Kelee meditation.

It is difficult to completely still your mind on command! The discipline of reaching stillness is an ongoing process. Do not let your frustrations deter you from practicing. Excellence takes time! Be kind and truthful when you grade the quality of your meditation.

3. *Contemplation.* This is the time to review how you are changing as your disharmony is released. Questions to ask are, *How do I feel about my practice? What changes am I noticing in my waking state?* I recommend students ponder how they feel and record their thoughts in a journal. As time passes, you will be amazed at how you have changed, with your journal an invaluable record of your growth.

27

Our mind
is the only private place
you will ever find.
And yes,
we all need one.
If you would like to find
your own peaceful space,
Kelee meditation
will show you the way.

Part Two

Kelee Meditation: The Meditation

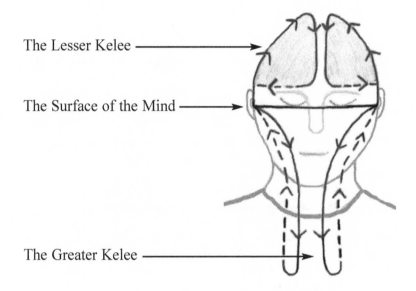

The Lesser Kelee ⎯⎯⎯⎯⎯⎯⎯⎯⎯

The Surface of the Mind ⎯⎯⎯⎯⎯

The Greater Kelee ⎯⎯⎯⎯⎯⎯⎯⎯

The Kelee and its Major Points of Reference

The Lesser Kelee ⟶

The Surface of the Mind ⟶

The Greater Kelee ⟶

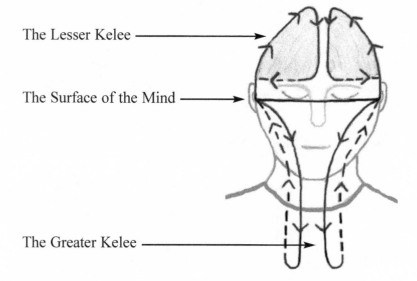

Kelee Meditation

Step One: *Approximately two minutes.*
Sit down, get comfortable, and begin relaxing your brain activity. Bring your conscious awareness to the top of your head and feel it as a horizontal plane of awareness relaxing down through both hemispheres of your brain to the surface of your mind. Be consciously relaxed, but not thinking.

Step Two: *Approximately three minutes.*
Relax and allow your awareness to drop below the surface of your mind into your greater Kelee to a still point within. The goal is to let go of sense consciousness and experience total stillness before returning to full consciousness.
Note: Before you drop from the surface your mind, set your biological clock to bring you back to complete awareness in about three minutes.

Step Three: *Approximately five minutes.*
Upon returning to the surface of your mind, reflect on what you noticed about your practice. Do not bolt into your day. Pace yourself.
Do your practice for ten minutes in the morning and evening to the best of your ability and get into the experience of your life. Allow the true nature of your being to unfold.
Recommendation: Keep a journal to write your experiences and record your progress. You think you will remember everything, but I can assure you, you will forget many subtle gems of wisdom about how you have grown.

*It is not
the shutting out
of thought
that you are trying
to achieve,
but an allowing
of stillness to happen.*

Part Three

Kelee Meditation: The Ins and Outs

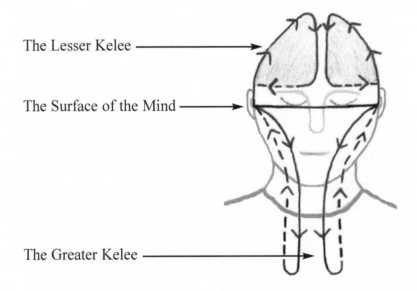

The Lesser Kelee ⎯⎯⎯⎯⎯⎯➤

The Surface of the Mind ⎯⎯⎯➤

The Greater Kelee ⎯⎯⎯⎯⎯➤

The Kelee and its Major Points of Reference

The Ins and Outs of Kelee Meditation

1. Be kind to yourself. Give yourself the gift of a clear mind—do your practice.

2. Do your practice for ten minutes in the morning and ten minutes in the evening. Allow the effects from Kelee meditation to manifest throughout your day.

3. Kelee meditation takes twenty minutes out of twenty-four hours, which is only one percent of your day. If you do not have one percent of twenty-four hours to cleanse the instrument running your whole life, how much self-control do you have?

4. If you are slow to wake up in the morning or too tired at bedtime, do your practice whenever possible, until you become accustomed to a morning and evening routine.

5. In **Step One** of Kelee meditation, relax your conscious awareness from the top of your head down to the surface of the mind without consciously thinking for about two minutes. Feel a distinction between a softened conscious awareness and the tension in the brain network. The goal is to have a relaxed conscious awareness without thoughts.

6. When your conscious awareness reaches the surface of the mind, do not worry if you do not drop below the surface into your greater Kelee; you are only experiencing your own resistance. When your resistance breaks down, you will drop. Be patient.

7. Set your biological clock for about three minutes before

you drop into your greater Kelee. This becomes automatic after the first few times.

8. The time you are in your Kelee is not the time to investigate what you see and experience! If you are thinking or spacing out, your conscious awareness cannot not be still. Stillness is the objective of Kelee meditation.

9. If you are falling asleep while meditating, you are either too tired or too relaxed. When your conscious awareness is too relaxed, it will spread out and wander. Refocus by pulling all of your awareness to a pinpoint within you. The sleep/stillness distinction takes time to master. Do Kelee meditation to the best of your ability.

10. Once you return to the surface of your mind, you can look back at what you remember about your practice. Keep a journal to record your experiences.

11. Do your practice even when you do not feel like it; this is when you need to do it the most.

12. The rewards received from Kelee meditation are experienced as mindfulness in your daily activities. Once again, total stillness in your practice is the goal, with enlightenment ultimately becoming your conscious way of being.

13. If you have not given Kelee meditation at least six months, you have not really given it a chance.

14. It is not unusual to feel a small drop in physical energy after beginning Kelee meditation, as you wean your

mind off hard, analytical, adrenaline-based energy. This feeling is transitory. After a short period of time your energy level will stabilize into an overall feeling of calmness, and you will have a new understanding of subtle energy.

15. When you begin to drop your walls, you may feel some emotional discomfort—this is known as "processing." Processing is what most people call a mood. When the discomfort or mood passes, you will not experience that particular dysfunction again.

16. When you are processing, be kind to yourself. You may want to sleep more than usual. This is normal. Give yourself a mental-health day, if you can. If not, pace yourself throughout your day.

17. From time to time you will experience physiological effects when processing, such as headaches, heartaches, nausea, low energy, or anxiety. If a button was linked with physical discomfort at the time it was formed, it will mimic the same response when it is being processed out. Any physical discomfort will cease when the dysfunction is released.
Everyone occasionally experiences physiological discomfort. Compartmentalized electrochemical dysfunction is at the nucleus of psychosomatic illness.

18. Sumadhi occurs when the space occupied by dysfunction is replaced by the true nature of your being. Sumadhi is a reward for your diligence—a potent, natural, euphoric feeling, stimulating an awareness of oneness with all things.

19. Mindfulness develops as your conscious awareness rises to a new level.

20. This practice will slow down the aging process. Each time you still your mind, degeneration declines, thereby allowing the physical body to rejuvenate. It is known that people who meditate are the longest-living people on the planet.

21. Efficiency will increase because your conscious awareness is not scattered, thereby naturally improving your ability to focus without distraction.

22. Depression will decrease. Worry, sadness, and degradation of oneself will plummet.

23. As negative, energy-draining programs are deleted, the immune system is free to function at an optimum power.

24. A deeper self-awareness enhances relationships at home and work with the ability to give from the heart without expecting anything in return.

25. Once you find the entrance to your soul and your greater Kelee, you will find your heart and never be lost again. As long as you continue to go within and be still each day, you will always be on your spiritual path.

26. The Three Disciplines of Kelee meditation are Meditation, Introspection, and Contemplation.

27. The Three P's of Kelee meditation are Practice, Persistence, and Patience.

What Next

Many people ask what order to read my books. After reading this book, if you would like a deeper understanding of Kelee meditation and the philosophy of the Kelee. I recommend reading *The Silent Miracle* the second book in this trilogy.

If you are interested in an understanding of the psychology of spirituality, I recommend reading *The Kelee*, the third book in this trilogy. This book brings a deeper understanding of the intimate connection between psychology and the mind.

Each book in this trilogy offers deeper levels of understanding of Kelee meditation and the philosophy of the Kelee.

If you would like to be inspired as to *why* it would be good to do Kelee meditation. *The Way is Within* presents gentle truths that begin to open your mind and lead you to a greater awareness of yourself. This book is an Oprah favorite. It has been featured in her magazine and on her website.

The second book, *The Mind and Self-Reflection* is a gentle introduction to the benefits of understanding the mind. It offers a new way to learn, and will change how you feel about yourself in a profoundly beautiful way.

I encourage you to enjoy them all!

Ron W. Rathbun